Table of Contents

Introduction

Cannabis oil is a special type of marijuana concentrate that has saved and improved countless lives. Cannabis oil is essentially pure THC or CBD which can be consumed in much larger doses than is possible by smoking, vaporizing, or ingesting raw cannabis flower.Cannabis oil, to be clear, is not the same thing as CBD oil. Do not buy CBD or hemp oils online. Such products are often produced from industrial grade hemp which lacks the critical anticancer THC cannabinoid. The industrial hemp used in these bogus medications is also often grown with harsh, inorganic chemical fertilizers as opposed to organic marijuana.Cannabidiol (CBD) is one of more than 100 unique "cannabinoid" compounds that are found in the oily resin of the cannabis plant. The sticky, gooey resin is concentrated on the dense clusters of cannabis flowers, commonly called "buds," which are covered by tiny, mushroom-shaped "trichomes." This is where the magic happens. Trichomes are specialized glandular structures that contain a treasure trove of oily, medicinal compounds, including CBD, tetrahydrocannabinol (THC), and various aromatic terpenes. Why does cannabis create these oily compounds? What does the resin do for the plant? The oily trichomes protect the plant from heat and ultraviolet radiation. The oil also has antifungal, antibacterial and insecticidal properties that deter predators. The stickiness of the resin provides another defensive layer by trapping bugs.

As it happens, the same oily resin that protects the health of the plant includes components that are beneficial for human health. CBD, a non-intoxicating compound, has shown promise in treating and managing the symptoms of a broad range of diseases. Ditto for THC, CBD's intoxicating cousin.CBD oil is extracted from the resinous trichomes of cannabis plants. There are many different cannabis "strains" or varietals. The amount of CBD present in the trichomes will depend on the particular variety of cannabis or hemp. Low resin industrial hemp, which is legally defined as cannabis with less than 0.3 percent THC by dry weight, has fewer trichomes – and therefore less oil – than high-resin cannabis varietals. But most high resin cannabis strains these days are THC-dominant with little CBD. So choosing the appropriate CBD-rich cannabis chemovar, a variety of cannabis defined by its chemical constituents, is key for extracting CBD oil.Trichomes are fragile structures that easily break off of the cannabis flower. Even rough handling is enough to shake off the trichomes. Making hashish or "kif" (hashish powder) involves manually removing the resinous trichomes by agitating the flower. Sometimes heat or pressure is applied to partially melt the trichomes together, turning the resin into a congealed slab, referred to as rosin, which can be smoked or ingested. In addition to the resinous trichomes concentrated on the flowers and to a lesser extent on the leaves of the cannabis plant, there are the tiny sessile trichomes, which dot the stalk, but these contain hardly any oil or CBD. (Shaped like tiny inverted commas, non-glandular hairs without oil also cover the plant's surface.) CBD is also absent in the roots or the seeds of cannabis and hemp. Companies that claim they derive CBD from hemp stalk or hemp seeds are making false claims.

What is CBD?

CBD is one of many cannabinoids (compounds) in the cannabis plant. Researchers have been looking at the possible therapeutic uses of CBD.Two of the compounds in marijuana are delta-9 tetrahydrocannabinol (THC) and CBD. These compounds have different effects.Until recently, THC was the best-known compound in cannabis. It is the most active constituent, and it has a psychological effect. It creates a mind-altering "high" when a person smokes it or uses it in cooking. This is because THC breaks down when a person applies heat and introduces it into the body. CBD, in contrast, is not psychoactive. It does not change a person's state of mind when they use it. However, it may produce significant changes in the body, and it is showing some significant medical benefits.Simply put, cannabis oil is the concentrated liquid extract of the marijuana plant, Cannabis sativa. Similar to other herbal extracts, the chemicals in cannabis oils vary depending on how the extract is made and what chemicals were in the plant to begin with. Cannabis plants produce thousands of compounds but the most well recognized belong to a class called cannabinoids. There are several cannabinoids but the two that are most well-known among consumers are THC (tetrahydrocannabinol) and CBD (cannabidiol).THC is the primary psychoactive compound in marijuana and it is what people are searching for when they want a product that gives them a "high."

Unlike THC, CBD isn't known to cause psychoactive effects, and is therefore attractive to those who want to avoid the high but who believe there are other benefits of CBD, said Sara Ward, a pharmacologist at Temple University in Philadelphia. [Healing Herb? Marijuana Could Treat These 5 Conditions] CBD products that don't contain THC fall outside the scope of the U.S. Drug Enforcement Agency's (DEA) Controlled Substances Act, which means CBD products are legal to sell and consume as long as they don't have THC. That's likely one of the reasons why CBD products, including CBD oil, are becoming more socially acceptable and increasingly popular. In 2016, Forbes reported that CBD products are expected to be a $2.2 billion industry by 2020.

What is cannabis oil?

Cannabis oils are extracts from cannabis plants. Unprocessed, they contain the same 100 or so active ingredients as the plants, but the balance of compounds depends on the specific plants the oil comes from. The two main active substances in cannabis plants are cannabidiol, or CBD, and delta-9 tetrahydrocannabinol, or THC. Oil extracted from hemp plants can contain a lot of CBD, while oil from skunk plants will contain far more THC. THC produces the high that recreational cannabis users seek, while oils for medical use contain mostly CBD.

Where does CBD come from?

CBD comes from the cannabis plant. People refer to cannabis plants as either hemp or marijuana, depending on how much THC they contain. The FDA note that hemp plants are legal under the Farm Bill, as long as they contain less than 0.3% THC. Over the years, marijuana farmers have selectively bred their plants to contain high levels of THC and other compounds that suited their interests. However, hemp farmers rarely modify the plant. CBD oil comes from these legal hemp plants.

How are CBD oils consumed?

The physiological effects of cannabinoids can vary widely from person to person, and also depend on how they're consumed. That lack of predictability is one of the reasons why cannabis oil is a challenging candidate for developing into a medicine, Ward told Live Science. "Two people may eat a brownie [made with cannabis oil] and one may absorb massive amounts of cannabinoids and the other may not," Ward said. "How long it takes to work and how long it stays in the system differs greatly." It's a little more uniform when the product is absorbed by smoking or vaping the oil, Ward said. But, "there are obvious concerns about smoking something." A 2007 review published in the journal JAMA Internal Medicine found that smoking marijuana resulted in similar declines in respiratory system health as smoking tobacco. A similar review published in 2014 in The American Journal of Cardiology found that marijuana smoke inhalation can increase the chances of heart attack or stroke. Neither review analyzed the effects of vaping cannabis oil alone, so it's unclear if it has the same health risks as smoking other marijuana products.

Why do people use cannabis oil?

People claim that cannabis oil can be used to treat a wide range of conditions, though evidence to back up these claims is often lacking. For example, according to Medical News Today, people use cannabis oil for conditions ranging from pain to acne; some even claim the oil can cure diseases like

Alzheimer's and cancer. (But again, there is no clinical evidence to support these claims.)

A review published in 2017 in the journal Frontiers in Pharmacology described how CBD may work to protect the hippocampus — the part of the brain responsible for several important functions, such as learning, memory and navigation — during times of stress, and may also help prevent brain-cell destruction that results from schizophrenia. Another 2017 review published in the journal Annals of Palliative Medicine

summarized a handful of studies
that suggest cannabis oils
containing THC or CBD, or both,
may help with chronic pain
management, but the mechanism
is unclear. Cannabis treatment in
people with certain forms of
epilepsy has been more promising.
The only FDA-approved cannabis-
based drug is Epidiolex, a CBD oral
solution for treating two rare and
severe forms of epilepsy. A recent
clinical trial found that Epidiolex
reduced convulsive seizures by
50% in children with Dravet

syndrome, a type of epilepsy, MedPage Today reported.

How To Make Cannabis Oil

First, gather your ingredients. You will need:

Three to four hours for the process from start to finish. 99.5% Isopropyl Alcohol. Use 2 gallons (7.57 liters) per pound or 2 cups (~500 ml) for an ounce of cannabis.

We also suggest chilling your alcohol in a freezer overnight. It will separate the trichomes from the flower more easily. Marijuana. Rick Simpson will use shake and trim to make topical solutions for skin afflictions. However, he insists that only the choicest, trichome-laden, cannabis indica colas should be used to make Canna Oil for treating cancer. The amount of cannabis oil that each strain can produce will vary, but one ounce of good organic marijuana will typically produce about three to four grams of oil. Rick Simpson's method works best with larger amounts of cannabis.

Next, gather your supplies. You will need:

Two stainless steel stock pots or food-grade plastic buckets.

Long wooden stirring spoon or 2×2 piece of chemical-free lumber.

Stainless steel rice cooker. Caution: A rice cooker with a non-stick

surface will leach chemicals into
your oil. Stick with
stainless steel only.

A common electric cooling fan and
extension cord.

Plastic funnels.

Coffee filters.

Empty clean plastic bottles.

Stainless steel measuring cup.

Coffee Warmer.

Large syringes.

Step 1

Place your weed of choice in a steel pot or food-grade bucket. Dampen the plant matter with chilled isopropyl alcohol (your solvent), and then crush the mixture with a wooden spoon or 2×2 for about five minutes.

Step 2

Add more alcohol until the plant matter is completely immersed. Again, crush and stir the mixture for a further five minute. The crushing action is technically called a "wash" because you are washing the trichomes from plant matter.

Step 3

Block the lip of the pot or bucket with a lid or your 2×2 and slowly pour the solvent into the second bucket. Try to keep as much of the marijuana plant matter in the first bucket for the next step. It's okay if some gets through—you're going to strain it later. But you want as much of the cannabis material left over in the first bucket as possible for the second round of washing.

Step 4

Pour more chilled alcohol into the first bucket until the plant matter is again immersed. Crush the cannabis with your wooden utensil for five more minutes. This step is known as the second wash.

Step 5

Again block the lip of the pot or bucket and slowly pour the solvent from the second wash into the bucket with the solvent from the first wash.

Step 6

Leave the solvent to sit while you recycle any leftover plant matter into your compost. Once converted to super soil, you can use it to grow more organic marijuana.

Step 7

Rinse out the first bucket.

Step 8

Place a coffee filter inside a plastic funnel and insert the funnel through the mouth of a small plastic bottle. The size of your straining container will depend on how much solvent you used in the first few steps. You can also use a number of smaller straining containers instead of trying to find one large container. Pour the mixture in the second bucket through the coffee filters to strain off any excess plant matter. Filter the solvent as many times as it takes to remove all the plant matter.

Step 9

Set up the rice cooker and the electric fan outside or in a well-ventilated area.

CAUTION: Make sure that there are no "sparks, open flames, or red-hot elements" in your workspace because the alcohol fumes that you will cook off in your rice cooker are highly flammable and toxic to inhale. Set up your fan so that it circulates air towards the vents on the bottoms of the rice cooker. See the picture above for a simple illustration of the cooker/fan arrangement. The reason for the fan is that it will prevent the alcohol fumes from condensing to a point where they can ignite.

Step 10

Fill the rice cooker as much as three-quarters full with your marijuana solvent mixture. Don't fill the cooker all the way up or it will boil over.The purpose of the next few steps is basically two fold: Separate the alcohol from the dissolved cannabis oil.

Decarboxylate the cannabis oil.

The vaporization (or boiling) point of isopropyl alcohol (the solvent you used in the first few steps) is around 181?. The vaporization point of cannabis oil is a little over 300?. The decarboxylation temperature for cannabis is in the low two hundreds (210-230?). Why do you need to know all these numbers? Because you have to maintain just the right temperatures so that your solvent boils off, your oil doesn't, and the leftover oil is decarboxylated. So why the rice cooker? Rice cookers are automatically set to maintain temperatures in the decarboxylation sweet spot. These temperatures are enough to get your solvent boiling but not enough to vaporize the oil. Crock pots often exceed 300? and a pot on the stove can be difficult to maintain a consistent low two-hundreds. Now that you know why you're using a rice cooker, we can move on to the actual separation process.

Step 11

Set the rice cooker to its highest
setting to boil off the alcohol
solvent. Be sure the fan is running
and is aimed at the rice cooker so
the alcohol fumes don't condense
and explode.

Step 12

As the liquid level in the rice
cooker drops, pour in any
remaining solvent but don't exceed
three-quarters full. This step
depends on how big your rice
cooker is and how much solvent
you produced in the first few steps

of the process. If you only have a small amount, you may not need to keep adding solvent.

Step 13

When you're done adding remaining solvent to the rice cooker, and the level in the cooker is reduced to about two inches, add ten to twelve drops of water to mix. The water will help the remaining solvent boil off and will cleanse the oil of solvent residue.

Step 14

Hold the rice cooker with oven mitts and swirl it's oily contents while the last traces of alcohol boil completely off.

Step 15

When the process is near completion, you will notice three things: The leftover oil will emit a crackling sound. The oil will begin to bubble (that's the source of the crackling sound). Steam will start to escape from the oil. It may look like smoke, but don't worry, it's dark steam. When those three criteria are satisfied, the separation process is almost done.

Step 16

Wait for the rice cooker to switch to the low setting and then turn it off.

Step 17

Let your fresh cannaoil mixture cool for about five minutes.

Step 18

Pour the mixture into a stainless steel measuring cup, and place the cup on a coffee warmer to completely remove any water remaining in the mixture. This process can take anywhere from a few minutes to an hour or more. It all depends on the terpenes and flavonoids found in the strain you used to make your oil. The terpenes and flavonoids can cause the oil on the coffee warmer to bubble for quite some time.

Step 19

 You know the water has been vaporized when all bubbling has ceased. Remove the measuring cup from the coffee warmer and set it aside to cool. Some oily residue will remain behind in the measuring cup and the rice cooker.

There are a number of options for dealing with these leftovers. You can soak it up with a piece of bread and consume it as medicine later. Keep in mind that the effects of edibles can take an hour or more to kick in. Be careful how much oil-soaked bread you consume. Wash the cup or the pot with a small amount of alcohol. This creates a hemp oil tincture that varies in medicinal value depending on the amount of oil the alcohol contains. You can use the isopropyl alcohol you used in the first few steps, but don't drink this mixture. Use the isopropyl alcohol tincture on your skin instead. For a tincture you can ingest, wash the rice cooker with a small amount of high-proof drinking alcohol like vodka or Everclear. Leave the leftovers in the rice cooker for the next time you make cannabis oil. Mixing the oils from different strains can have many beneficial medicinal effects.

Step 20

After the oil has cooled, draw the warm mixture up into large needleless syringes and allow the mixture to cool into a thick grease like substance that you can easily squeeze out of the syringe. Place the syringe in a cup of hot water if you have trouble squeezing it out after it has cooled. If you're not going to use your cannabis oil right away, store it in a dark bottle with a lid or a stainless steel container and place that container in a dark, cool place. This keeps air and sunlight from damaging your valuable creation and helps the oil maintain its medical potency for a long time. "At first, it may seem daunting for some to try to produce their own medicine," Rick Simpson says. But in reality, the process is extremely simple. Simpson also strongly suggests mixing your favorite varieties of good indica-dominant buds to make your own custom marijuana miracle potions. Place a small amount of loose tobacco in the rice cooker and heat until the oil is absorbed. The cannabis oil reduces many of the harmful properties contained in the tobacco.

Cannabis Oil Applications

Topical Uses

Apply the oil directly to skin cancers, cover with a bandage, and reapply and rebandage every four days until the cancer disappears. Continue the treatment for two more weeks to completely heal any cancer cells which could remain. "I have never seen a skin cancer return if my instructions are followed," Rick says. You can also try mixing your cannabis oil with coconut oil and use the concoction for general daily skin health. This mix of cannabis and coconut oil can turn your skin green for a bit depending on how well you made the cannabis oil. Don't worry though, it will wash off. To keep this green tinge from becoming a problem, you could apply the oil at night and then scrub it off in the morning when you shower.

Edible Uses

Cannabis oil is much more concentrated than regular

cannabis products like the bud you smoke. For that reason, it's best to start small and work your way up from there. Rick Simpson suggests 1 gram (or 1 ml) of homemade cannabis oil as a full dose. One gram of cannabis oil looks like a pile of about 16 to 8 grains of dry short-grain rice. But again, before you run out and down a gram of cannabis oil, Rick recommends starting small.In general, he says, it takes new users about 90 days to work up to ingesting the full treatment without getting dysfunctionally high. That's why

Simpson starts new patients off with a serving size that looks like half a dry grain of rice. That may seem tiny and inconsequential, but remember, cannabis oil is quite a bit more concentrated than other cannabis products.

Start off taking this half-a-dry-grain-of-rice serving three times a day. An easy schedule to follow is:

First thing in the morning with breakfast

In the afternoon after lunch

About an hour before you go to sleep

Follow this dosage for four days, then double the dosage to the size of a full grain of rice for the next four days (see the chart above). Rick typically doubles the dosage for patients every four days until they reach the full amount. Taking the full dose head on without titrating (building up to it) will certainly not kill you. Indeed, some of his patients report enjoying the full dose right off the bat. And Simpson has seen brand new patients with no 420 fears take the full dose first thing. Many of these patients are declared completely cancer-free just one month after beginning the full dose. According to Simpson, "The name of the game," in terms of actually ingesting the dose, "is to simply get the oil into the patient's body in the easiest and most pleasant way possible."

Dosage Methods

One of the many nice things about cannabis oil is that you can take it in a variety of ways. Below, we describe some of the most common (and easiest) ways to consume cannabis oil.

Ingest It Directly

The simplest way to consume your cannabis oil is to place it directly on top of your tongue and let it dissolve. You can also place it under your tongue and let it dissolve down your throat. If you don't like the taste, you can also smear the oil on a piece of bread or in between two pieces of fruit (we like banana) to avoid the taste. You could also try mixing it in your favorite drink to make it easier to consume. Ingesting the cannabis oil in this way should give you the strong kind of 11-Hydroxy-THC body high with an onset that can take up to two hours. If you're familiar with edibles, this is the same thing.

Place It Under Your Tongue (Sublingual)

Another way to consume your cannabis oil is to dab the cannaoil under your tongue and let it dissolve into your bloodstream through your sublingual artery. This method produces effects a little bit faster than ingesting it. The results will be akin to a heady marijuana tincture high.

Vaporize It

You can also vaporize cannabis oil in a vape pen. This is an extremely easy way to take your cannabis oil with you wherever you go. Simply fill up the vape pen's chamber with your homemade oil, and you're ready to go anytime.

Dab It

Another great way to consume cannabis oil is to dab it on a rig like a concentrate. Dabbing a bit of cannabis oil is one of the quickest ways to feel the effects. When you vaporize the cannabis oil, as you do when you dab, the vapor is absorbed much more quickly into your bloodstream and reaches your brain much sooner than it would if you ingest it. You will, of course, need a special dabbing rig, but the initial outlay of money is well worth it for the fast-acting high or pain relief you can achieve.

Smoke It

And, of course, you can always rely on the old tried-and-true method of consuming cannabis products: you can smoke it. How do you smoke an oil? Like this. For a truly out-of-this-world experience, we highly recommend first glazing a joint of your favorite marijuana strain in cannabis oil. Then, cover the whole thing in kief crystals. The resulting combination is a stone cold recreational high! Just be careful. This much ganja goodness in one place can take you on a truly transcendental trip.

Benefits and Uses of CBD Oil (Plus Side Effects)

Cannabidiol is a popular natural remedy used for many common ailments. Better known as CBD, it is one of over 100 chemical compounds known as cannabinoids found in the cannabis or marijuana plant, Cannabis sativa (1Trusted Source). Tetrahydrocannabinol (THC) is the main psychoactive cannabinoid found in cannabis, and causes the sensation of getting "high" that's often associated with marijuana.

However, unlike THC, CBD is not psychoactive. This quality makes CBD an appealing option for those who are looking for relief from pain and other symptoms without the mind-altering effects of marijuana or certain pharmaceutical drugs. CBD oil is made by extracting CBD from the cannabis plant, then diluting it with a carrier oil like coconut or hemp seed oil. It's gaining momentum in the health and wellness world, with some scientific studies confirming it may ease symptoms of ailments like chronic pain and anxiety. Here are health benefits of CBD oil that are backed by scientific evidence.

Can Relieve Pain

Marijuana has been used to treat pain as far back as 2900 B.C. More recently, scientists have discovered that certain components of marijuana, including CBD, are responsible for its pain-relieving effects. The human body contains a specialized system called the endocannabinoid system (ECS), which is involved in regulating a variety of functions including sleep, appetite, pain and immune system response. The body produces endocannabinoids, which are neurotransmitters that bind to cannabinoid receptors in your nervous system. Studies have shown that CBD may help reduce chronic pain by impacting endocannabinoid receptor activity, reducing inflammation and interacting with neurotransmitters. For example, one study in rats found that CBD injections reduced pain response to surgical incision, while another rat study found that oral CBD treatment significantly reduced sciatic nerve pain and inflammation. Several human studies have found that a combination of CBD and THC is effective in treating pain related to multiple sclerosis and arthritis. An oral spray called Sativex, which is a combination of THC and CBD, is approved in several countries to treat pain related to multiple sclerosis. One study of 47 people with multiple sclerosis examined the effects of taking Sativex for one month. The participants experienced improvements in pain, walking, and muscle spasms. Still, the study didn't include any control group and placebo effects cannot be ruled out. Another study found that Sativex significantly improved pain during movement, pain at rest and sleep quality in 58 people with rheumatoid arthritis.

Could Reduce Anxiety and Depression

Anxiety and depression are common mental health disorders

that can have devastating impacts on health and well-being. According to the World Health Organization, depression is the single largest contributor to disability worldwide, while anxiety disorders are ranked sixth. Anxiety and depression are usually treated with pharmaceutical drugs, which can cause a number of side effects including drowsiness, agitation, insomnia, sexual dysfunction and headache. What's more, medications like benzodiazepines can be addictive and may lead to substance abuse. CBD oil has shown promise as a treatment for both depression and anxiety, leading many who live with these disorders to become interested in this natural approach. In one Brazilian study, 57 men received either oral CBD or a placebo 90 minutes before they underwent a simulated public speaking test. The researchers found that a 300-mg dose of CBD was the most effective at significantly reducing anxiety during the test. The placebo, a 150-mg dose of CBD, and a 600-mg dose of CBD had little to no effect on anxiety. CBD oil has even been used to safely treat insomnia and anxiety in children with post-traumatic stress disorder. CBD has also shown antidepressant-like effects in several animal studies. These qualities are linked to CBD's ability to act on the brain's receptors for serotonin, a neurotransmitter that regulates mood and social behavior.

Can Alleviate Cancer-Related Symptoms

CBD may help reduce symptoms related to cancer and side effects related to cancer treatment, like nausea, vomiting and pain.

One study looked at the effects of CBD and THC in 177 people with cancer-related pain who did not experience relief from pain medication. Those treated with an extract containing both compounds experienced a significant reduction in pain compared to those who received only THC extract. CBD may also help reduce chemotherapy-induced nausea and vomiting, which are among the most common chemotherapy-related side effects for those with cancer. Though there are drugs that help with these distressing symptoms, they are sometimes ineffective, leading some people to seek alternatives. A study of 16 people undergoing chemotherapy found that a one-to-one combination of CBD and THC administered via mouth spray reduced chemotherapy-related nausea and vomiting better than standard treatment alone. Some test-tube and animal studies have even shown that CBD may have anticancer properties. For example, one test-tube study found that concentrated CBD induced cell death in human breast cancer cells. Another study showed that CBD inhibited the spread of aggressive breast cancer cells in mice. However, these are test-tube and animal studies, so they can only suggest what might work in people. More studies in humans are needed before conclusions can be made.

May Reduce Acne

Acne is a common skin condition that affects more than 9% of the population. It is thought to be caused by a number of factors, including genetics, bacteria, underlying inflammation and the overproduction of sebum, an oily secretion made by sebaceous glands in the skin. Based on recent scientific studies, CBD oil may help treat acne due to its anti-inflammatory properties and ability to reduce sebum production. One test-tube study found that CBD oil prevented sebaceous gland cells from secreting excessive sebum, exerted anti-inflammatory actions and prevented the activation of "pro-acne" agents like inflammatory cytokines. Another study had similar findings, concluding that CBD may be an efficient and safe way to treat acne, thanks in part to its remarkable anti-inflammatory qualities (25Trusted Source). Though these results are promising, human studies exploring the effects of CBD on acne are needed.

Might Have Neuroprotective Properties

Researchers believe that CBD's ability to act on the endocannabinoid system and other brain signaling systems may provide benefits for those with neurological disorders. In fact, one of the most studied uses for CBD is in treating neurological disorders like epilepsy and multiple sclerosis. Though research in this area is still relatively new, several studies have shown promising results. Sativex, an oral spray consisting of CBD and THC, has been proven to be a safe and effective way to reduce muscle spasticity in people with multiple sclerosis. One study found that Sativex reduced spasms in 75% of 276 people with multiple sclerosis who were experiencing muscle spasticity that was resistant to medications. Another study gave 214 people with severe epilepsy 0.9–2.3 grams of CBD oil per pound (2–5 g/kg) of body weight. Their seizures reduced by a median of 36.5%. One more study found that CBD oil significantly reduced seizure activity in children with Dravet syndrome, a complex childhood epilepsy disorder, compared to a placebo. However, it's important to note that some people in both these studies experienced adverse reactions associated with CBD treatment, such as convulsions, fever and fatigue. CBD has also been researched for its potential effectiveness in treating several other neurological diseases. For example, several studies have shown that treatment with CBD improved quality of life and sleep quality for people with Parkinson's disease. Additionally, animal and test-tube studies have shown that CBD may decrease inflammation and help prevent the neurodegeneration associated with Alzheimer's disease. In one long-term study, researchers gave CBD to mice genetically predisposed to Alzheimer's disease, finding that it helped prevent cognitive decline.

Could Benefit Heart Health

Recent research has linked CBD with several benefits for the heart and circulatory system, including the ability to lower high blood pressure. High blood pressure is linked to higher risks of a number of health conditions, including stroke, heart attack and metabolic syndrome. Studies indicate that CBD may be able to help with high blood pressure. One recent study treated nine healthy men with one dose of 600 mg of CBD oil and found it reduced resting blood pressure, compared to a placebo. The same study also gave the men stress tests that normally increase blood pressure. Interestingly, the single dose of CBD led the men to experience a smaller blood pressure increase than normal in response to these tests . Researchers have suggested that the stress- and anxiety-reducing properties of CBD are responsible for its ability to help lower blood pressure. Additionally, several animal studies have demonstrated that CBD may help reduce the inflammation and cell death associated with heart disease due to its powerful antioxidant and stress-reducing properties. For example, one study found that treatment with CBD reduced oxidative stress and prevented heart damage in diabetic mice with heart disease.

Several Other Potential Benefits

CBD has been studied for its role in treating a number of health issues other than those outlined above.

Though more studies are needed, CBD is thought to provide the following health benefits:

Antipsychotic effects: Studies suggest that CBD may help people with schizophrenia and other mental disorders by reducing psychotic symptoms.

Substance abuse treatment: CBD has been shown to modify circuits in the brain related to drug addiction. In rats, CBD has been shown to reduce morphine dependence and heroin-seeking behavior.

Anti-tumor effects: In test-tube and animal studies, CBD has demonstrated anti-tumor effects. In animals, it has been shown to prevent the spread of breast, prostate, brain, colon and lung cancer.

Diabetes prevention: In diabetic mice, treatment with CBD reduced the incidence of diabetes by 56% and significantly reduced inflammation.

Quitting smoking and drug withdrawal

A 2013 pilot study found that smokers who used inhalers containing CBD smoked fewer cigarettes than usual and stopped craving nicotine. This suggests that CBD may help people quit smoking. A 2018 study found that CBD helped reduce cravings during withdrawal from tobacco because of its relaxing effect. Authors of a

2015 review found evidence that specific cannabinoids, such as CBD, may help people with opioid addiction disorders. The researchers noted that CBD reduced some symptoms associated with substance use disorders. These included anxiety, mood-related symptoms, pain, and insomnia.

Epilepsy

After years of research into the safety and effectiveness of CBD oil for treating epilepsy, the FDA approved the use of Epidiolex, a purified form of CBD, in 2018.

They approved it for treating the following in people aged 3 years and over:

Lennox-Gastaut syndrome

Dravet syndrome

These rare forms of epilepsy involve seizures that are difficult to control with other types of medication. Scientists are beginning to understand how CBD prevents seizures without the sedating side effects of medications used previously. Synthetic drugs are not yet available that target the endocannnabinoid system as CBD does.

Alzheimer's disease

Numerous studies have looked at the effect of CBD on Alzheimer's disease. In 2014, a rodent study showed that CBD might help people retain the ability to recognize familiar faces. People with Alzheimer's can lose this ability. One 2019 review found that CBD might help slow the onset and progress of Alzheimer's disease. More research is underway to understand the dosage better. Some scientists believe a treatment involving both THC and CHD may be more effective.

Other neurological symptoms and disorders

Research suggests that CBD may also help treat complications linked to epilepsy, such as neurodegeneration, neuronal injury, and psychiatric diseases. A 2012 study found that CBD may produce effects similar to those of certain antipsychotic drugs and that the compound may provide a safe and effective treatment for people with schizophrenia. However, further research is necessary.

Are There Any Side Effects?

Though CBD is generally well tolerated and considered safe, it may cause adverse reactions in some people.

Side effects noted in studies include:

Diarrhea

Changes in appetite and weight

Fatigue

CBD is also known to interact with several medications. Before you start using CBD oil, discuss it with your doctor to ensure your safety and avoid potentially harmful interactions. This is especially important if you take medications or supplements that come with a "grapefruit warning." Both grapefruit and CBD interfere with cytochromes P450 (CYPs), a group of enzymes that are important to drug metabolism. One study performed on mice showed that CBD-rich cannabis extracts have the potential to cause liver toxicity. However, some the mice in the study were force-fed extremely large doses of the extract .

Conclusions

CBD oil has been studied for its potential role in easing symptoms of many common health issues, including anxiety, depression, acne and heart disease. For those with cancer, it may even provide a natural alternative for pain and symptom relief. Research on the potential health benefits of CBD oil is ongoing, so new therapeutic uses for this natural remedy are sure to be discovered. Though there is much to be learned about the efficacy and safety of CBD, results from recent studies suggest that CBD may provide a safe, powerful natural treatment for many health issues. If you're interested in trying CBD, you can purchase many products online,

including gummies, oils, and
lotions.